Emergency Paediatric

Contents

Subject	Section	Page

Emergency Paediatric First Aid is published by: **Nuco Training Ltd**

WHAT IS PAEDIATRIC FIRST AID?

In all of our lives, whether at work, home or at play, it is essential that we all know how to assist a child or infant who is sick, or has been injured.

Paediatric First Aid, as the term implies, is the initial treatment given to a child or infant who is injured or sick, prior to professional medical assistance arriving and taking over from you.

By reading this manual, it will not make you a doctor, paramedic or nurse, but by applying common sense and some basic life support skills, as well as providing care and confidence in your treatment for the casualty, you will learn skills that will enhance their well-being and in some very serious cases, possibly save their life.

Your prompt, safe and effective treatment could make a difference between life and death.

As a Paediatric First Aider, your priorities for the casualty fall into the following categories:

PRESERVE life

ALLEVIATE suffering

PREVENT the condition from worsening

PROMOTE recovery

For instance, if your casualty is suffering major blood loss as a result of a serious cut, then you can **preserve life** by offering treatment immediately and not waiting for professional help to sort it out for you. If you do nothing, then your casualty could bleed to death.

We can **alleviate suffering** by making the casualty more comfortable, reducing their pain levels and offering lots of care and attention.

We can **prevent further illness or injury** by applying a secure sterile dressing on the injured part in order to control the blood loss and prevent the risk of infection.

We can **promote recovery** by treating the casualty for shock and ringing for an ambulance.

DEFINITION OF PAEDIATRIC

The term paediatric refers to children and infants (babies).

The Resuscitation Council UK (RCUK) and European Resuscitation Council (ERC) defines an infant (baby) as being under 1 year old. They define a child as being from 1 year old through to 18 years old. If the rescuer is in any doubt as to the age of the casualty, then they should adopt paediatric protocols.

ACTS AND REGULATIONS

For some, you may have a responsibility in the workplace for first aid. Should this be the case then you must be aware of legislation that ensures employers provide a duty of care, along with a first aid provision for their employees, as well as non-employees and contractors visiting their premises.

THE HEALTH AND SAFETY AT WORK ACT 1974

This Act, also abbreviated to HSWA, HASWA or HASAWA, is an Act of the Parliament of the United Kingdom that currently defines the fundamental structure and authority for the encouragement, regulation and enforcement of workplace health, safety and welfare within the United Kingdom.

The Act defines general duties on employers, employees, contractors, suppliers of goods and substances for use at work, persons in control of work premises, and those who manage and maintain them, and persons in general.

THE MANAGEMENT OF THE HEALTH AND SAFETY AT WORK REGULATIONS 1999

These Regulations generally make more explicit what employers are required to do to manage health and safety under the Health and Safety at Work Act. Like the Act, they apply to every work activity, including the provision of first aid. The main requirement for employers is to carry out a risk assessment. Employers with five or more employees need to record the significant findings of the risk assessment. Risk assessment should be straightforward in a simple workplace such as a typical office.

THE HEALTH AND SAFETY (FIRST AID) REGULATIONS 1981 (1982 IN NORTHERN IRELAND)

The Health and Safety (First-Aid) Regulations 1981 require employers to provide adequate and appropriate equipment, facilities and personnel to ensure their employees receive immediate attention if they are injured or taken ill at work.

PAEDIATRIC FIRST AID PROVISION

You should liaise with management and other First Aider's to ensure:

- **There is an adequate number of Paediatric First Aiders, First Aiders and Emergency First Aiders in place**
- **Appropriate equipment, kits and facilities are available**
- **A system is in place for incident and accident reporting**

It is vital that a risk assessment of first aid needs is conducted to ensure that the correct level of provision is made.

Where the risk assessment identifies the need for people to be available for rendering first aid, then the employer should ensure that they are provided in sufficient numbers and at appropriate locations to enable first aid to be administered without delay, should the occasion arise.
Guidance on the Regulations for employers was introduced in October 2013 (L74 – Third edition).

The following table will guide you in ensuring that you have sufficient numbers of trained first aid personnel at your place of work.

1. From your risk assessment, what degree of hazard is associated with your work activities	2. How many employees do you have?	3. What first aid personnel do you need?	4. What injuries and illnesses have previously occurred in your workplace	5. Have you taken account of the factors below that may affect your first aid provision?
Low-hazard eg offices, shops, libraries	Fewer than 25	At least **1 appointed person**	• Ensure any injuries or illness that may occur can be dealt with by the First Aiders you provide • Where First Aiders are shown to be unnecessary, there is still a possibility of an accident or sudden illness, so you may wish to consider providing qualified First Aiders	• Inexperienced workers or employees with disabilities or particular health problems • Employees who travel a lot, work remotely or work alone • Employees who work out-of-hours • Premises spread out across buildings/floors • Workplace remote from the emergency services • Employees working at sites occupied by other employers • Planned & unplanned absences of first-aider/appointed person • Members of the public who visit the workplace
	25 - 50	At least **1 EFAW** trained First Aider		
	More than 50	At least **1 FAW** trained First Aider for every 100 employed (or part thereof)		
Higher hazard eg light engineering and assembly work, food processing, warehousing, extensive work with dangerous machinery or sharp instruments, construction, chemical manufacture	Fewer than 5	At least **1 appointed person**		
	5 - 50	At least **1 EFAW** or **FAW** trained First Aider, depending on the type of injuries that may occur		
	More than 50	At least **1 FAW** trained First Aider for every 50 employed (or part thereof)		

Information supplied by Health & Safety Executive. The Health and Safety (First-Aid) Regulations 1981 L74 (Third edition 2013)

FIRST AID CONTAINERS

The minimum level of first aid equipment is a suitably stocked and properly identified first aid container. Every employer should provide, for each work site, at least one first aid container supplied with a sufficient quantity of first aid materials suitable for the particular circumstances.

There is no mandatory list of items to be included in a first aid container. The decision on what to provide, will be influenced by the findings of the first aid needs assessment. As a guide, where work activities involve low hazards, a minimum stock of first aid items might be:

- **A guidance leaflet**
- **20 individually wrapped plasters**
  (Assorted sizes)
- **2 sterile eye pads**
- **2 triangular bandages**
  (Individually wrapped and preferably sterile)
- **6 medium sterile wound dressings**
  (Individually wrapped and un-medicated)
- **2 large sterile wound dressings**
  (Individually wrapped and un-medicated)
- **At least 3 pairs of disposable gloves**
- **6 safety pins**

This is a suggested contents list only.

The contents of first aid containers should be examined frequently and restocked soon after use.

PERSONAL PROTECTIVE EQUIPMENT (PPE)

Employers should supply adequate PPE stored near to the first aid supplies. Such equipment could include hand sanitiser, face masks, safety glasses, ear protection, hi-vis vests and flashlights. Employers should also advise First Aiders on what PPE should be worn in which circumstances, ensuring that the First Aider's safety is the priority.

ADDITIONAL FIRST AID MATERIALS AND EQUIPMENT

The needs assessment may indicate that additional materials and equipment are required, for example scissors, burns dressings, adhesive tape, disposable aprons and individually wrapped moist wipes. They may be kept in the first aid container if there is room, or stored separately.

If mains tap water is not readily available for eye irrigation, at least a litre of sterile water or sterile normal saline (0.9%) in sealed, disposable containers should be provided. Once the seal has been broken, containers should not be kept for re-use. Containers should not be used beyond their expiry date.

It is recommended that tablets and medicines should not be kept in the first aid container.

First Aid at Work does not include giving tablets or medicines to treat illness.

The view of the Health and Safety Executive (HSE), is that the administration of medication by a First Aider is not part of a First Aid at Work training course, but you can assist an individual in taking it, if it is their own medication.

However, the one exception is heart attacks. Therefore, for heart attack management, you can assist a casualty in taking one aspirin tablet (300mg) and ask them to chew it slowly, providing you are confident that the casualty is not allergic to it. If you are in any doubt, then you MUST NOT administer it. Aspirin MUST NOT be administered to anyone under the age of 16.

ACCIDENT AND INCIDENT REPORTING

Irrespective of the severity of the accident or incident, it is vital that all such occurrences be reported and filed by the employer.

Anyone can complete the accident book, and this book must comply with Data Protection legislation.

The accident book should be used as a useful reference for the purpose of ensuring that, where reasonably practicable, the same incident can be prevented from happening again.

An accident book can be purchased at most good book shops, or online from many first aid supply shops.

The information that should be recorded includes:

- **The date, time and place of the incident**
- **Name and job of the injured or ill person**
- **Details of the injury/illness and what first aid was given**
- **What happened to the casualty immediately afterwards?** (e.g. went back to work, went home, went to hospital)
- **Name and signature of the person reporting the incident**
- **The information must be kept in accordance with the Data Protection Act 2018**

Where the incident is of a severe nature, then the employer must comply with RIDDOR 2013.

RIDDOR is the law that requires employers, and other people in control of work premises, to report and keep records of:

- **Work-related accidents which cause death**
- **Work-related accidents which cause certain serious injuries (reportable injuries)**
- **Diagnosed cases of certain industrial diseases**
- **Certain 'dangerous occurrences' (incidents with the potential to cause harm)**

There are also special requirements for gas incidents.

Reporting certain incidents is a legal requirement. The report informs the enforcing authorities (HSE, local authorities and the Office for Rail Regulation (ORR)) about deaths, injuries, occupational diseases and dangerous occurrences, so they can identify where and how risks arise, and whether they need to be investigated.

Please visit www.hse.gov.uk/riddor/ for full details of what is reportable.

RESPONSIBILITIES

A Paediatric First Aider has a number of responsibilities when dealing with an incident.

It is paramount that the incident is dealt with confidently and safely. The safety for all is important, including you, the casualty and any bystanders.

You must manage the incident and take control of the situation until professional medical help arrives and takes over. A bystander can be a great benefit to you, particularly if they are qualified in first aid, so don't be afraid to summon help.

A bystander can make a telephone call, get a first aid kit, return with the defibrillator if you have one, manage the crowd and traffic, and generally support you.

Your responsibilities can be broken up into the following categories:

- Arrival at the scene
- Dealing with casualties
- Casualty communication
- Contacting the emergency services
- Prioritise the first aid treatment
- Clearing up process and infection control

ARRIVAL AT THE SCENE

Make the area safe and gather as much information about the incident as you can. The history of the incident and any casualty information about their illness or injury could help you decide your course of initial treatment.

Ensure you have help at hand.

You are almost certain to be feeling nervous and anxious yourself, but be as confident as you can, and take control of the situation.

DEALING WITH CASUALTIES

- **Prioritise your treatment, particularly if you have multiple casualties**
- **Ensure safety for all**
- **Protect against contamination**
- **Be calm and confident**
- **Ensure that the appropriate emergency services have been called for**

CASUALTY COMMUNICATION

Irrespective of the severity of the incident, your casualty could be in a state of shock and confusion. Therefore, your communication skills are critical in gaining their trust.

The groups that are most likely to be affected are children, the elderly, hearing impaired, visually impaired and non-English speaking casualties.

- **Be honest about their condition, without exaggerating it**
- **Be careful of what you say which could distress them further**
- **Maintain eye contact when talking to them, and be aware of your body language. Their body language could tell you a lot about their condition**
- **Take your time when talking to them, particularly for the vulnerable groups such as the elderly and children**
- **Allow your casualty to explain how they are feeling. It could help you make a diagnosis enabling you to offer the right treatment**
- **In respect of their injury, avoid medical terms that they may not understand**
- **Explain to the parents or guardians what is being done**
- **Provide a child with a comforter such as a toy or their blanket**

CONTACTING THE EMERGENCY SERVICES

As soon as you have identified the extent of the injury, then it may be necessary to contact the emergency services.

They can be contacted by dialling 999 or 112.

They will require vital information about the condition of the casualty so that the call can be prioritised.

Activate the speaker function on the phone to aid communication with the ambulance service.

They will also require specific details about the location of the incident. It is imperative that you have the full details of where you are, particularly if the premises are large and have multi-floors or other buildings to consider. Your bystander could manage this for you by meeting the emergency services and guiding them to the incident.

Only dial 999 if it is necessary and consider other services such as the Police and Fire, dependent on the incident.

Remember **LIONEL** when making this call:

L **Location**

I **Incident**

O **Other services**

N **Number of casualties**

E **Extent of injuries**

L **Location - repeat**

PRIORITISE YOUR FIRST AID TREATMENT

- **Breathing** – deal with casualties who are not breathing normally first
- **Bleeding** – deal with any major bleeding and treat the casualty for shock
- **Burns/breaks** – treat burns and immobilise any bone injuries
- **Other conditions** – treat appropriately

There are many conditions that could be deemed as life-threatening which require medication, such as diabetes, asthma and anaphylaxis. Where possible, you can assist your casualty by offering them their own medication if they have it with them.

Remember your priorities. Ensure that their airway remains open and that they are breathing normally for themselves.

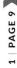

THE CLEARING UP PROCESS AND INFECTION CONTROL

You must minimise the risk of infection from the outset when dealing with any incident. This applies to you, the casualty, and any bystanders. Similarly, when the casualty has been treated it is vital that all soiled dressings etc, are disposed of correctly.

- **Wash your hands and wear disposable gloves**

- **Avoid coughing and sneezing over the wound, and avoid touching it**

- **Dispose of all soiled dressings, including gloves, in an appropriately marked (orange/yellow) plastic bag**

- **Dispose of sharp items, including syringes and needles, in a purpose made sharps bin and dispose of it appropriately. It may mean taking it to your local hospital for correct disposal**

Rescuers should take appropriate safety precautions where feasible, especially if the casualty is known to have a serious infection such as tuberculosis (TB), severe acute respiratory distress syndrome (SARS) or coronavirus (COVID-19).

During any outbreak of a highly infectious condition, protective precautions for the rescuer are essential.

When confronted with any emergency situation, you need to take **SHAPE!**

SAFETY AND PROTECTION

You must ensure the safety for all. Ensure you are adequately protected against the risk of infection and any other adverse element such as chemicals and gases

HAZARDS

Be aware of potential hazards such as traffic, chemicals, fire, gas, electricity etc

ASSESS THE SITUATION

Before rushing in to deal with an incident, you must assess the situation that you are confronted with

PRIORITISE

Ensure you prioritise the injuries, particularly if you have multiple casualties

ENVIRONMENT

Pay attention to the environment around you, and do not take risks. Jumping into water to save a drowning victim is not a good idea if you can't swim!

Irrespective of the incident you are confronted with, you must carry out an initial assessment of the situation including your casualty.

This is popularly known as the primary survey.

The contents of this survey can be remembered easily by using the mnemonic **DR ABC**.

D Dangers

The area must be safe before you offer your casualty any treatment. Safe for you primarily, not forgetting any bystanders and of course your casualty.

Failing to do this could result in you having more casualties to deal with, which could include yourself!

R Response

Approach the casualty, ideally from their feet.

This reduces the risk of the casualty hyper-extending their neck should they be responsive.

If they are responsive, ascertain the extent of their injury and deal with it appropriately.

If they are not responsive, then:

- Gently stimulate the child and ask loudly, 'Are you all right?'

- An infant can be stimulated by rubbing the soles of their feet with your finger

- Do not shake infants, or children with suspected cervical spine injuries

- Use their name when talking to them

If they respond by answering or moving:

Leave them in the position in which you find them (provided they are not in further danger).

Check their condition, reassess them regularly and move on to your secondary assessment (page 15).

NB: If you need to make a telephone call, always endeavour to take the child or infant with you. Ideally they should not be left alone.

If there is no response at all, they must be deemed as being unresponsive.

If you are on your own, you should shout for help. Ideally, you should never leave your casualty on their own.

A bystander can be a great benefit to you such as:

- **Calling for an ambulance**

- **Managing crowds and hazards**

- **Fetching the first aid kit and defibrillator if you have one**

- **Consoling relatives and friends**

- **Helping you if they are trained to do so**

- **Cleaning up**

- **A support for you**

A Airway

Turn the child/infant onto their back and open their airway using the head tilt and chin lift manoeuvre:

- Place your hand on their forehead and gently tilt their head back. Be very careful not to over extend this movement with an infant
- With two fingertips under the point of their chin, lift the child's chin. Use one finger for an infant

In either case, do not push on the soft tissues under the chin as this may block the airway.

B Breathing

Look, listen and feel for normal breathing for no more than 10 seconds.

Look for chest movement

Listen at their mouth for breath sounds

Feel for air on your cheek

In the first few minutes after cardiac arrest, a casualty may be barely breathing, or taking infrequent, noisy, gasps. This is often termed agonal breathing or gasping, and must not be confused with normal breathing. If you have any doubt whether breathing is normal, act as if it is not normal and prepare to commence CPR.

C CPR for a non-breathing casualty

If their breathing is not normal or absent:

- Send your bystander immediately to call for an ambulance and to return with a defibrillator, if one is available, whilst you commence CPR without delay (See page 20)

If you have no bystander, then:

- Carefully remove any obvious airway obstruction
- Give 5 initial rescue breaths followed by 1 minute of CPR
- Call for an ambulance
- Continue with CPR

If you are able to, activate the speaker function on your phone to aid communication between you and the emergency services.

The casualty who is **unresponsive** and not **breathing normally** is in cardiac arrest and requires CPR.

Immediately following cardiac arrest blood flow to the brain is reduced to virtually zero, which may cause seizure-like episodes that may be confused with epilepsy.

You should be suspicious of cardiac arrest with any casualty that presents seizure like symptoms and carefully assess whether they are breathing normally.

If they are breathing normally:

- If your casualty is unresponsive, but breathing normally, with no evidence of major physical trauma, they should be placed in the recovery position (see page 16)

- Ask your bystander to summon an ambulance. If you are on your own, then make this call yourself taking the casualty with you if it's possible. Maintain an open airway by holding them in the recovery position. If it's not possible, place them in the recovery position in order to maintain an open airway before leaving them

- **Upon your return ensure that they are in the recovery position and monitor their breathing until the emergency services take over from you.** Should they stop breathing normally, then start CPR (see page 20)

If you are unsure about the extent of the injury, then try to make a diagnosis based upon the signs that you can see, the symptoms that the casualty is feeling and the history, before placing them in the recovery position (see page 16).

SECONDARY ASSESSMENT

As soon as you have completed your primary survey, and you have established that your casualty is breathing normally, you must then move on to the secondary assessment in order to determine the extent of their injury or illness, irrespective of whether they are responsive or not.

In order to make a diagnosis of their condition, there are three key factors to consider. By making this diagnosis correctly, it should determine the treatment you offer them. In all cases, your priority is to maintain an open airway and to ensure that they are breathing normally.

History

- Ask your casualty or bystanders what happened
- Examine the environment for obvious signs relating to the incident
- Ask your casualty about their condition. Do they have their own medication? Has it happened before? Where does it hurt? How painful is it?
- Ask the casualty their name. Is there any family present that could answer the questions about their condition?

Signs

- What can you see in respect of the injury or condition?
- Use all your other senses. What can you smell, hear and feel?

Symptoms

This is how the casualty will be feeling, ask them how they are feeling.

- **Communication is very important to ascertain the extent of their injury/illness**
- **Continue to question their well-being throughout your assessment as they may have deteriorated which may influence your decision on the appropriate treatment**

THE RECOVERY POSITION FOR A CHILD

If your casualty is unresponsive, but breathing normally, with no evidence of major physical trauma then your priority is to ensure that their airway is not compromised in any way and that it remains open. Rather than leaving them on their back, or in a slumped position, then an effective way of achieving this is to place them in the recovery position.

Whilst the casualty remains in this position, it will allow vomit to drain from the mouth and prevent them from rolling onto their back should you have to leave them.

1 **Remove the casualty's glasses, if present**

2 **Kneel beside the casualty and make sure that both their legs are straight**

3 **Place the arm nearest to you out at a right angle to their body, elbow bent with the hand palm-up. Do not force the arm, let it fall naturally, but close to this position**

4 **Bring the far arm across the chest, and hold the back of the hand against their cheek nearest to you**

5 **Grab hold of the far leg with your other hand, and raise the knee so that their foot is kept to the floor. This will be your lever for rolling them over**

6 **Keeping their hand pressed against their cheek, pull on the far leg to roll them towards you onto their side with their head supported all the way**

7 Tilt the head back to make sure that the airway remains open

8 Adjust the upper leg so that both the hip and knee are bent at right angles

9 If you have a bystander available to you, then this is the time to send them to call for an ambulance ensuring they have all the appropriate information, and in particular, the condition of the casualty

10 If you have no bystander, you must call for an ambulance yourself

If they have to be kept in the recovery position for **more than 30 minutes** turn them to the opposite side to relieve the pressure on the lower arm.

You must continue to monitor their breathing whilst waiting for the emergency services to take over. If they stop breathing normally, then you must call the emergency services with an update and commence CPR immediately.

It will also be worth monitoring and noting other changes such as colouration of the skin, their temperature and responsiveness levels.

THE RECOVERY POSITION FOR AN INFANT

If the infant is unresponsive, but breathing normally, with no evidence of major physical trauma then your priority is to ensure that their airway is not compromised in any way and that it remains open.

Rather than leaving them on their back, an effective way of achieving this is to place them in the recovery position.

Hold the infant in your arms with their head facing downwards and towards you so that you can monitor their airway, their breathing and their general condition.

If their condition deteriorates in any way, then it is vital to update the emergency services.

It is important to keep them with you at all times, particularly when contacting the emergency services.

Whilst the casualty remains in this position, it will allow vomit to drain from their mouth and maintain an open airway.

If their breathing stops or it is not normal, then:

- **Send your bystander immediately to call for an ambulance whilst you commence CPR without delay**

If you have no bystander, then:

- **Carefully remove any obvious airway obstruction**
- **Give 5 initial rescue breaths followed by 1 minute of CPR**
- **Call for an ambulance**
- **Continue with CPR**

THE RESPIRATORY SYSTEM

Our ability to breathe is thanks to our respiratory system which is made up primarily of our airways and our lungs.

We are able to breathe in and out spontaneously providing we have air to breathe and the airways are open.

COMPOSITION OF AIR

Air breathed in

- Nitrogen - 78%
- Oxygen - 21%
- Argon and other gases - 1%

When we breathe in the diaphragm contracts and flattens, the ribs are elevated, and as negative pressure is produced in the chest cavity, there is increased pressure in the abdomen. This draws air into the lungs to equalise the pressure.

We exhale when the diaphragm relaxes and the chest wall and lung tissue returns to their original size.

Respiration is achieved through the mouth, nose, trachea, lungs, and diaphragm. Oxygen enters the respiratory system through the mouth and the nose. The oxygen then passes through the larynx (where speech sounds are produced) and the trachea which is a tube that enters the chest cavity. In the chest cavity, the trachea splits into two smaller tubes called the bronchi. Each bronchus then divides again forming the bronchioles. These bronchial tubes lead directly into the lungs where they divide into many smaller tubes which connect to tiny sacs called alveoli. The average adult's lungs contain about 600 million of these spongy, air-filled sacs that are surrounded by capillaries. The inhaled oxygen passes into the alveoli and then enters the capillaries (diffusion) into the arterial blood which is taken back to the heart for circulating around the body.

Meanwhile, the waste-rich blood from the veins releases its carbon dioxide into the alveoli. The carbon dioxide follows the same path out of the lungs when you breathe out.

Approximately 25% of the available oxygen in each breath is used, as our body can only cope with so much each time we breathe in.

Carbon dioxide and other non-essential gases are breathed out, and the whole process is repeated approximately:

30-40 times for an infant under the age of 1		
25-35 times for a child	1-2 years of age	
25-30 times for a child	2-5 years of age	
20-25 times for a child	5-12 years of age	
10-20 times for someone > 12 years of age		

The Respiratory System

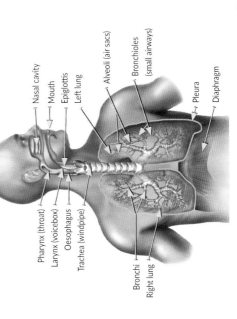

- Nasal cavity
- Mouth
- Epiglottis
- Left lung
- Alveoli (air sacs)
- Bronchioles (small airways)
- Pleura
- Diaphragm
- Pharynx (throat)
- Larynx (voicebox)
- Oesophagus
- Trachea (windpipe)
- Bronchi
- Right lung

Cardiopulmonary resuscitation (CPR) is an emergency procedure which is attempted in an effort to return life to a child or infant who is not breathing normally for themselves.

This procedure combines chest compressions with rescue breaths. The chest compression replaces the heart's ability to pump oxygenated blood around the body, particularly the vital organs such as the brain.

Rescue breathing provides the casualty, who is unable to breathe normally for themselves, valuable oxygen that is transported around the body in the bloodstream by the chest compressions.

Without oxygen, brain damage can occur within three minutes. Therefore, your immediate action is paramount.

Referring back to Primary Survey, ie: DR ABC, you will have established that your casualty is not breathing normally.

Your immediate action now is to send your bystander to call the emergency services for an ambulance, ensuring they have the correct information, with particular reference that your casualty is not breathing normally.

- **Carefully remove any airway obstruction**

- **Give 5 initial rescue breaths**

- **Give 30 chest compressions followed by a further 2 rescue breaths**

- **Repeat the sequence 30-2**

If you don't have a bystander, then you must administer 5 initial breaths, followed by 1 minute of CPR (approximately 2 cycles of 30 chest compressions followed by 2 breaths) before contacting the emergency services yourself.

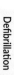

Continue with CPR (30-2) until the emergency services take over from you, your casualty recovers* or you become too exhausted to continue.

CHILD

For rescue breath technique - see page 21

For chest compression technique - see page 23

INFANT

For rescue breath technique - see page 22

For chest compression technique - see page 24

* Recovery means that they start to show signs of life i.e. they wake up or, start moving or, open their eyes **and** they start to breathe normally for themselves.

Defibrillation

If you have an Automated External Defibrillator (AED) available to you, you should immediately unpack it, attach the pads, switch it on and follow the voice prompts. (Please see pages 25-29 for further information).

TECHNIQUE FOR GIVING RESCUE BREATHS FOR A CHILD OVER 1 YEAR:

- Ensure head tilt and chin lift
- Pinch the soft part of their nose closed with the index finger and thumb of your hand on their forehead

- Open their mouth a little, but maintain the chin lift
- Take a breath and place your lips around their mouth, making sure that you have a good seal

- Blow steadily into their mouth over 1 second, sufficient to make the chest rise visibly. This is the same time period as in adult practice
- Maintaining head tilt and chin lift, take your mouth away and watch for their chest to fall as air comes out
- Take another breath and repeat this sequence four more times. Identify the effectiveness by seeing that their chest has risen and fallen in a similar fashion to the movement produced by a normal breath

TECHNIQUE FOR GIVING RESCUE BREATHS FOR AN INFANT:

- Ensure a neutral position of the head (as an infant's head is usually flexed when on their back and face up (supine), this may require some extension) and apply chin lift

- Take a breath and cover the mouth and nose of the infant with your mouth, making sure you have a good seal. If both the nose and mouth cannot be covered in the older infant, then attempt to seal only the infant's nose or mouth with your mouth (if the nose is used, close the lips to prevent air escape and vice versa)

- Blow steadily into their mouth over 1 second, sufficient to make the chest rise visibly. This is the same time period as in adult practice

- Maintain head position and chin lift, take your mouth away, and watch for their chest to fall as air comes out

- Identify the effectiveness by seeing that their chest has risen and fallen in a similar fashion to the movement produced by a normal breath

For both infants and children, if you have difficulty achieving an effective breath, the airway may be obstructed:

- Open their mouth and remove any visible obstruction. Do not perform a blind finger sweep

- Ensure that there is adequate head tilt and chin lift but also that the neck is not over extended

- Make up to 5 attempts to achieve effective breaths. If this is still unsuccessful, move on to chest compressions

TECHNIQUE FOR GIVING CHEST COMPRESSIONS FOR CHILDREN AGED OVER 1 YEAR:

- Place the heel of one hand on the lower half of the breastbone (sternum)
- Lift the fingers to ensure that pressure is not applied over their ribs
- Position yourself vertically above their chest and, with your arm straight, compress the sternum to depress it by at least one-third of the depth of the chest, which is approximately 5cms, and at a speed of 100-120 compressions per minute. For larger children, or for small rescuers, this may be achieved more easily by using both hands with the fingers interlocked

After giving 30 chest compressions, give 2 rescue breaths.

Repeat the sequence of 30:2.

Continue with CPR (30:2) until the emergency services take over from you, your casualty recovers* or you become too exhausted to continue.

* Recovery means that they start to show signs of life i.e. they wake up, or start moving, or open their eyes **and** they start to breathe normally for themselves.

TECHNIQUE FOR GIVING CHEST COMPRESSIONS FOR INFANTS:

- Place the tips of 2 fingers in the centre of the breastbone (sternum)

- Compress the sternum to depress it by at least one-third of the depth of the chest which is approximately 4cms

- Release the pressure completely, then repeat at a rate of 100-120 compressions per Minute

- After giving 30 chest compressions, give 2 rescue breaths

- Repeat the sequence of 30:2

- Continue with CPR (30:2) until the emergency services take over from you, your casualty recovers* or you become too exhausted to continue

* Recovery means that they start to show signs of life i.e. they wake up, or start moving, or open their eyes **and** they start to breathe normally for themselves.

DEFIBRILLATION WITH AN AED

In the rare event a child needs defibrillating, follow these guidelines as detailed on Pages 25 – 28 but pay particular attention to Page 29 where specific information can be found on paediatric pads.

The resuscitation procedure for a child will be the same as detailed earlier.

If your casualty is wearing jewellery that may come into contact with the pads, then it must be removed.

When the AED arrives, you must immediately unpack it and prepare to fix the pads to the casualty. If you have trained help, then allow them to continue with CPR until you are ready. If not, then stop CPR and unpack it yourself.

The majority of pads will be clearly marked on where they should be fixed. Depending on the make and model of the AED, the pads will generally come as two separate pads. Some will come as a single pad. Ensure that the film that is protecting the sticky pads is removed.

If your casualty has a pacemaker fitted, then ensure that the pads are placed at least 10cms away from it.

Do not place the pads directly on top of it. A pacemaker should be clearly identifiable, from a scar or what appears to be a small plate under the skin.

Most AED pads are labelled left and right, or carry a picture of the placement. It does not matter if these pads are reversed. What is important is that should they be placed the wrong way round, they must be left in place because the adhesive may well be removed or compromised if you swap them around.

In respect of switching the AED on, they will vary from one AED to another. Some will switch themselves on as soon as the lid is removed or opened. Others will have a button to press to switch it on.

It is important that you familiarise yourself with the AED you have.

All AED's will have a voice prompt and it is important that you follow these prompts.

Some AED's will also have a screen giving you the commands. This can be a very useful aid for those who are hard of hearing.

It is important from here on in to follow these prompts as soon as the pads are connected and the AED is switched on.

The AED will need to analyse the heart's rhythm. You will be prompted to ensure that no-one is touching the casualty, including yourself. Anyone touching the casualty could have an adverse effect on detecting the correct rhythm of your casualty's heart.

Dependent on the model you have, analysis will automatically happen, or you may have to push the 'Analyse' button.

You have to take control of the situation and move people away from the casualty.

Your next prompt could be to shock the casualty. Your AED may do this automatically, or you may have to press the 'Shock' button.

Again, manage the situation and ensure that no-one is touching the casualty.

Keep following the prompts from the AED.

If you are prompted to commence CPR, then quality CPR is important.

Ensure that you compress the chest at the right depth (dependent on age), and at the right speed of 100-120 chest compressions per minute.

In essence you must continue with CPR until the AED tells you to stop to either analyse the casualty's heart rhythm, or it decides that a shock should be given.

Under the current Resuscitation guidelines, you will be administering CPR for two minutes before the AED will prompt you to stop in order for it to analyse the heart's rhythm.

You must continue to follow the prompts until professional medical help takes over from you, your casualty recovers, or you become too exhausted to continue. Recovery will mean that your casualty shows signs of regaining responsiveness, such as coughing, opening their eyes, speaking or moving purposefully AND they start to breathe normally for themselves. To ensure they are breathing normally, conduct a breathing check.

If you are confident that they are breathing normally, place them in the recovery position with the pads attached and connected to the AED.

You must continue to monitor their breathing until professional medical help arrives and takes over from you.

PAEDIATRIC DEFIBRILLATION

The protocol for paediatric defibrillation is the same as that for an adult.

Most manufacturers are able to offer you specially modified pads for children, that means you can use the same AED for adults and children. However, what it is important to know are the differences between adults, children and infants in respect of your Basic Life Support procedures. This section deals with those differences.

The term paediatric refers to children and infants (babies).

A child is deemed as being aged 1 year old through to 18 years old, and an infant being aged under 1 year old.

Many manufacturers refer to children as being from the age of 1 to 8. Any child that is older than 8 years of age should be treated as an adult, and the adult protocols for CPR and defibrillation should be adopted.

Most manufacturers will have specially adapted pads to accommodate a child.

The pads for children are generally smaller. When they are connected to the AED, the device will recognise them and administer the appropriate electric shock, which is generally a reduced charge.

Defibrillation is not recommended for infants unless the manufacturer of the AED you have has specially adapted pads that can be connected. You must check with your supplier to see if pads are available.

If you have an incident to deal with that involves a child or infant, then you should carry out a primary survey as defined in section 2.

THE CHAIN OF SURVIVAL

It is critical that you follow this chain when you are dealing with a casualty who is not breathing normally.

Early recognition and call for help

Recognise those at risk of cardiac arrest, and call for help in the hope that early treatment can prevent arrest.

Early CPR

Start CPR to buy time until medical help arrives.

Early defibrillation

Defibrillators give an electric shock to re-organise the rhythm of the heart.

Defibrillation within 3–5 minutes of cardiac arrest can produce survival rates as high as 50–70%.

Each minute of delay to defibrillation reduces the probability of survival to hospital discharge by 10%.

Post-resuscitation care

Provide professional help in order to restore the quality of life.

SEIZURES

WHAT IS EPILEPSY?

Epilepsy is a condition that affects the brain. When someone has epilepsy, it means they have a tendency to have epileptic seizures.

Anyone can have a one-off seizure, but this doesn't always mean they have epilepsy. Epilepsy is usually only diagnosed if someone has had more than one seizure, and doctors think it is likely they could have more.

Epilepsy can start at any age and there are many different types. Some types of epilepsy last for a limited time and the person eventually stops having seizures. But for many people epilepsy is a life-long condition.

WHAT ARE EPILEPTIC SEIZURES?

A seizure happens when there is a sudden burst of intense electrical activity in the brain. This causes a temporary disruption to the way the brain normally works.

The result is an epileptic seizure.

There are many different types of seizure. What happens to someone during a seizure depends on which part of their brain is affected. During some types of seizure, the person may remain alert and aware of what's going on around them, and with other types they may lose awareness. They may have unusual sensations, feelings, or movements. Or they may go stiff, fall to the floor and jerk.

WHAT CAUSES EPILEPSY?

Possible causes of epilepsy include:

- Stroke
- **A brain infection, such as meningitis**
- **Severe head injury**
- **Problems during birth which caused the baby to get less oxygen**

But in over half of all people with epilepsy, doctors don't know what caused it. Some may have a family history of epilepsy, suggesting that they may have inherited it.

Tonic-clonic seizures are the type of seizure most people recognise.

Someone having a tonic-clonic seizure goes stiff, loses responsiveness, falls to the floor and begins to jerk or convulse. They may go blue around the mouth due to irregular breathing. Sometimes they may lose control of their bladder or bowels, and bite their tongue or the inside of their mouth.

HOW TO HELP IF YOU SEE SOMEONE HAVING A TONIC-CLONIC SEIZURE

Do:

- Protect them from injury (remove harmful objects from nearby)
- Cushion their head
- Look for an epilepsy identity card or identity jewellery – it may give you information about their seizures and what to do
- Time how long the jerking lasts
- Aid breathing by gently placing them in the recovery position once the jerking has stopped
- Stay with the them until they are fully recovered
- Be calmly reassuring

Don't:

- Restrain their movements
- Put anything in their mouth
- Try to move them unless they are in danger
- Give them anything to eat or drink until they are fully recovered
- Attempt to bring them round

Call for an ambulance if:

- You know it is their first seizure or
- The jerking continues for more than five minutes or
- They have one tonic-clonic seizure after another without regaining responsiveness between seizures or
- They are injured during the seizure or
- You believe they need urgent medical attention

FOCAL SEIZURES

This type of seizure can also be called a partial seizure. Someone having a focal seizure may not be aware of their surroundings or what they are doing. They may have unusual movements and behaviour such as plucking at their clothes, smacking their lips, swallowing repeatedly or wandering around.

How to help if you see someone having a focal seizure.

Do:

- Guide them away from danger (such as roads or open water)
- Stay with them until recovery is complete
- Be calmly reassuring
- Explain anything that they may have missed

Don't:

- Restrain them
- Act in a way that could frighten them, such as making abrupt movements or shouting at them
- Assume they are aware of what is happening, or what has happened
- Give them anything to eat or drink until they are fully recovered
- Attempt to bring them round

Call for an ambulance if:

- You know it is their first seizure or
- The seizure continues for more than five minutes or
- They are injured during the seizure or
- You believe they need urgent medical attention

AIRWAY OBSTRUCTION

When a foreign body enters the airway the child reacts immediately by coughing in an attempt to expel it. A spontaneous cough is likely to be more effective and safer than any manoeuvre you might perform. However, if coughing is absent or ineffective, and the object completely obstructs the airway, the child will become asphyxiated rapidly. Active interventions to relieve choking are therefore required only when coughing becomes ineffective, but they then must be commenced rapidly and confidently.

The majority of choking events in children occur during play or whilst eating, when a carer is usually present. Events are therefore frequently witnessed, and interventions are usually initiated when the child is responsive.

Choking is characterised by the sudden onset of respiratory distress associated with coughing, gagging, or stridor, a high-pitched wheeze. Similar signs and symptoms may also be associated with other causes of airway obstruction, such as laryngitis or epiglottitis, which require different management.

Suspect choking caused by a foreign body if:

- The onset was very sudden
- There are no other signs of illness
- There are clues to alert you, for example a history of eating or playing with small items immediately prior to the onset of symptoms

General signs of choking

- Witnessed episode
- Coughing or choking
- Sudden onset
- Recent history of playing with or eating small objects

Ineffective coughing

- Unable to vocalise
- Quiet or silent cough
- Unable to breathe
- Cyanosis
- Decreasing level of responsiveness

Effective cough

- Crying or verbal response to questions
- Loud cough
- Able to take a breath before coughing
- Fully responsive

RELIEF OF CHOKING

Safety and summoning assistance

Safety is paramount. You should avoid placing yourself in danger and consider the safest action to manage the choking child:

- If the child is coughing effectively, then no external manoeuvre is necessary. Encourage the child to cough, and monitor continuously

- If the child's coughing is, or is becoming, ineffective, shout for help immediately and determine the child's responsive level

Responsive child who is choking

- If the child is still responsive but has absent or ineffective coughing, give back blows

- If back blows do not relieve choking, give chest thrusts to infants or abdominal thrusts to children

  These manoeuvres create an 'artificial cough' to increase pressure in the chest cavity and dislodge the foreign body.

Back blows for an infant

- Support the infant in a head-downwards, prone position, to enable gravity to assist the removal of the foreign body
- If you are seated or kneeling, you should be able to support the infant safely across your lap

  - Support the infant's head by placing the thumb of one hand at the angle of the lower jaw, and one or two fingers from the same hand at the same point on the other side of the jaw
  - Do not compress the soft tissues under their jaw, as this will worsen the airway obstruction
  - Deliver up to 5 sharp back blows with the heel of one hand in the middle of the back between the shoulder blades
  - The aim is to relieve the obstruction with each blow rather than to give all 5

Back blows for a child

- Back blows are more effective if the child is positioned head down
- A small child may be placed across the rescuer's lap as with an infant

  - If this is not possible, support the child in a forward-leaning position and deliver the back blows from behind

If back blows fail to dislodge the object, and they are still responsive, use chest thrusts for infants or abdominal thrusts for children. Do not use abdominal thrusts for infants.

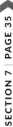

Chest thrusts for infants:

- Turn them on to their back so they are facing up. With your free arm, support their head and ensure that the airway remains open without too much extension

- Support them down your arm, which is placed down (or across) your thigh

- Identify the landmark for chest compression which is the centre of their chest on the lower part of their sternum

- Deliver up to 5 chest thrusts. These are similar to chest compressions, but sharper in nature and delivered at a slower rate

- The aim is to relieve the obstruction with each thrust rather than to give all 5

Abdominal thrusts for children over 1 year:

- Stand or kneel behind them and place your arms under their arms and encircle their torso

- Clench your fist and place it between the navel and the bottom of their breastbone

- Grasp this hand with your other hand and pull sharply inwards and upwards

- Repeat up to 4 more times

- The aim is to relieve the obstruction with each thrust rather than to give all 5

Repeat the sequence of up to 5 back blows followed by up to 5 chest thrusts for an infant, up to 5 abdominal thrusts for a child, until the obstruction is relieved or they become unresponsive.

NB: If the obstruction is still there after 1 cycle of back blows and abdominal/chest thrusts, you must summon an ambulance immediately. If you have to make this call yourself, then take the child/infant with you. Continue with your treatment of up to 5 back blows followed by up to 5 abdominal or chest thrusts.

If the object is expelled successfully you must seek medical advice, particularly if chest thrusts or abdominal thrusts have been given.

Unresponsive child or infant who is choking

- If the choking child is, or becomes, unresponsive place them on a firm, flat surface

- Call for an ambulance immediately. Send your bystander to make this call if you have one

- Do not leave the child or infant on their own if you have to make this call yourself

- Start CPR immediately (see page 20), but before each rescue breath attempt, look for any visible obstruction and remove it. If one is seen, make an attempt to remove it with a single finger sweep

Do not attempt blind or repeated finger sweeps

These can impact the object more deeply into the airway and cause injury.

The circulatory system is our body's transport system for two fluids, namely, blood and lymph.

For the purposes of first aid we will focus on the transport of blood, also known as the cardiovascular system.

This system consists of the heart and blood vessels, which supply our body, and in particular, our vital organs such as the brain and heart, with blood containing oxygen and nutrients to keep them healthy.

Our heart is a hollow muscular pump, about the size of your fist, with two pairs of chambers. These chambers collect blood flowing back from our body after depositing the oxygen and nutrients, before being pumped back to the lungs to collect more oxygen so that the cycle of transportation can continue.

The adult heart beats approximately 60 - 80 times every minute and pumps approximately six litres of blood around our body every minute.

The blood vessels within this system are:

- **Arteries**

  Deliver oxygenated blood from the heart to the body, with the exception of the pulmonary artery which carries de-oxygenated blood from the heart to the lungs

- **Veins**

  Carry the de-oxygenated blood back to the heart

- **Capillaries**

  Much smaller vessels that form a link between the arteries, veins and body tissue to allow the transfer of oxygen and nutrients to the body and the waste products to be removed

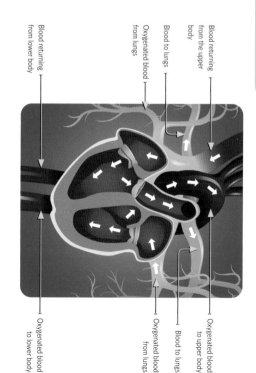

Blood returning from the upper body

Blood to lungs

Oxygenated blood from lungs

Blood returning from lower body

Oxygenated blood to upper body

Blood to lungs

Oxygenated blood from lungs

Oxygenated blood to lower body

Blood is made up of:

- **Plasma**

  The fluid component of the blood of which 90% is water

- **Platelets**

  Help to block the blood flow by clotting

- **Red cells**

  Transport the oxygen via the haemoglobin

- **White cells**

  Manufacture antibodies and fight infection and bacteria

HYPOVOLAEMIC SHOCK

There are a number of reasons why this system could fail, including blood loss, failure of the heart, poor circulation, a fall in blood pressure and the lack of oxygen contained within the body.

Other conditions include poisoning, vomiting, infection, burns and injury to the spinal cord, but this is by no means the definitive list.

As a First Aider, there are a number of things we can do for our casualty such as to stop the bleeding and to take pressure off the heart. This will be covered later, but one of your main concerns should be that hypovolaemic shock will set in very quickly if you don't react quickly enough, and shock can be a killer!

Hypovolaemic shock is best described as a failure or collapse of the circulatory system when the arterial blood pressure is too low to provide an adequate blood supply to the tissues.

Signs and symptoms of hypovolaemic shock

- Ashen coloured skin (grey/blue)
- Clammy and cold skin to touch
- Feeling of sickness and thirst
- Their breathing will be rapid and shallow

Treatment of hypovolaemic shock

- Deal with the injury or condition
- Make them comfortable and lay them down
- Raise both legs providing it does not compromise their injuries further
- Keep them warm and maintain their response levels by talking to them
- Call for an ambulance
  - Monitor their response and breathing
  - Do not allow them to eat or drink as it may affect their well-being and it could compromise further treatment

FAINTING

Fainting is a sudden, usually temporary, brief loss of responsiveness generally caused by insufficient oxygen in the brain.

The signs and symptoms are the same as shock with the exception that the pulse rate is slower.

A casualty who has fainted will generally make a rapid recovery and feel fine very quickly.

TREATMENT FOR SOMEONE WHO FEELS FAINT

- Help them to the floor and lie them down
- Raise and support their legs
- Offer them plenty of fresh air
- Sit them up gradually
- Comfort and reassure them

TREATMENT FOR SOMEONE WHO HAS FAINTED

If a person faints and does not regain responsiveness within one or two minutes, you should put them into the recovery position, monitor their breathing and medical assistance should be sought.

A wound can be best described as a type of injury in which the skin is torn, cut or punctured (an open wound), or where a blunt force created a contusion (a bruise).

In first aid there are 6 types of wounds that you should be familiar with:

INCISION
Clean cut as with a knife blade

LACERATION
Rough tear as with barbed wire

ABRASION
Scrape as with a gravel rash

CONTUSION
A blunt blow causing bruising

PUNCTURE
A stabbing type wound

VELOCITY
Gunshot wound

When a blood vessel is torn or severed, blood loss and shock cause the blood pressure to fall and the injured vessels will contract at the site of injury.

Platelets and proteins come into contact with the injured site and plug the wound.

This clotting process begins within ten minutes if the loss of blood is brought under control.

BLEEDING IS CLASSIFIED BY THE TYPE OF BLOOD VESSEL THAT IS DAMAGED.

Arterial Pumps from the wound with the heartbeat

Venous Gushes from the wound or pools at the site

Capillary Oozing at the site of injury

Once you have completed your initial casualty assessment for prioritising your treatment, you must follow the guidelines for personal protection and hygiene control before you begin to treat the casualty.

Treatment for the control of bleeding

- Put on disposable gloves

- Expose and examine the wound

- Apply direct pressure with your fingers or palm, preferably over a sterile dressing or non-fluffy clean pad (you can ask your casualty to apply this pressure)

- Elevate and support the injured part for wounds that are not catastrophic

- Help the casualty to lie down and raise the legs if you suspect shock

- Secure the dressing with a bandage large enough to cover the wound

- If blood seeps through this dressing, remove both the dressing and bandage and apply pressure to the bleed with a new dressing

- Secure the new dressing with a bandage once the bleeding is under control

- Support the injured limb with a sling or bandaging if appropriate, providing the casualty allows you to do so

- Monitor their response levels and call for an ambulance

CATASTROPHIC BLEEDING

If you are unable to stop the bleeding because of the severity, then you will need to apply direct pressure continually and then pack the wound with haemostatic dressings, or apply a tourniquet.

If you have neither, then you must continue to apply direct pressure and consider making an improvised tourniquet. It is imperative that you call for an ambulance immediately for a severe, or catastrophic bleed.

To summarise the treatment for catastrophic bleeding

- Do apply direct pressure to the wound

- Do use a haemostatic dressing or tourniquet

- Do not apply indirect pressure to proximal pressure points

- Do not elevate an extremity

Fortunately, the vast majority of businesses would never have to deal with a catastrophic bleed in a first aid situation at work. For most First Aiders, blood loss can be controlled by following the guidelines as detailed to the left of this text.

> **It must be emphasised that further training is required for First Aiders in respect of using haemostatic dressings or tourniquets.**
>
> **Please speak to your training provider.**

EMBEDDED OBJECTS

If during your examination of the wound you see an embedded object such as a piece of glass, then you must leave it in place and dress around it.

Your aim is to stop the bleeding, but care must be taken not to put any direct pressure on the embedded object.

| Check the wound for anything embedded | Apply dressing and pressure to either side of the object | Apply a larger sterile dressing over the top | Secure the bandage | Elevate the injured limb | Treat for shock |

BLEEDING FROM ORIFICES

Signs, symptoms and causes

Site	Appearance	Cause
Mouth	Bright red, frothy, coughed up.	Bleeding in the lungs.
	Vomited blood, red or dark reddish brown.	Bleeding in the stomach.
Ear	Fresh bright-red blood.	Injury to ear, perforated eardrum.
	Thin, watery blood.	Head injury.
Nose	Fresh bright red blood.	Ruptured blood vessel in nostril.
	Thin, watery blood.	Skull fracture.
Anus	Fresh bright-red blood.	Injury to anus or lower bowel.
	Black tarry, offensive smelling stool.	Injury to upper bowel.
Urethra	Urine with red or smoky appearance and occasional clots.	Bleeding from the bladder, kidneys.
Vagina	Either fresh or dark blood	Menstruation, miscarriage, disease or injury to the vagina or womb.

TREATMENT

- Treat the cause where possible using sterile dressings
- Treat the casualty for shock
- Monitor their condition, particularly their breathing
- Call 999/112 for an ambulance
- Lay them injured side down where possible
- Do not try to plug the wound, but cover it with a sterile dressing
- Offer them plenty of reassurance
- Pay attention to the casualty's modesty and dignity, particularly if they are bleeding from the anus or vagina

AMPUTATIONS

Any part of the body that has been severed will need immediate hospital treatment.

There is almost certain to be severe blood loss, and your aim as an Emergency First Aider is to control the bleeding, treat for shock and to protect and transport the amputated body part to hospital with the casualty.

Your prompt and effective treatment may just allow the amputated part to be stitched back successfully with micro-surgery.

Signs and symptoms

- Bleeding
- Shock
- Severe pain in the majority of cases
- An open wound
- Amputated body part

Treatment

- Ensure that the area is safe. Turn off machinery etc, that may have caused the accident
- Control the loss of blood by applying direct pressure with a sterile, non-fluffy dressing
- Treat the casualty for shock
- Reduce the risk of cross-infection by wearing gloves
- Call 999/112 for an ambulance
- Wrap the amputated part in plastic such as cling-film
- Wrap it further in a cloth
- Submerge the wrapped and protected part in ice. It is important that the severed part does not make direct contact with the ice. Mark the package clearly with the casualty's name and ensure that it is transported to hospital with the casualty
- Protect and maintain an open airway
- Monitor their breathing. Be prepared to resuscitate the casualty if they stop breathing normally

MINOR CUTS AND GRAZES

Cuts and grazes are some of the most common injuries.

Minor cuts and grazes (where only the surface layer of skin is cut or scraped off) may bleed and feel slightly painful, but the affected area will normally scab over and heal quickly.

However, if the cut is in an area that is constantly moving, such as your knee joint, it may take longer to heal.

Depending on how deep the cut is and where it is on your body, a scar may remain once the cut has healed.

Deeper cuts may damage important structures below the skin such as nerves, blood vessels or tendons.

However, grazes that remove the deeper layers of skin are rare.

Most cuts and grazes can be easily treated by cleaning them thoroughly and covering them with a plaster or dressing.

Please bear in mind that hypoallergenic plasters are available should your casualty have an allergy to ordinary plasters.

SEEK MEDICAL HELP IF ANY OF THE BELOW APPLY:

You think there is damage to deeper tissues: signs include numbness (indicating injury to a nerve), blood spurting from the wound or bleeding that does not stop after five minutes of continuous firm pressure.

The wound is at risk of becoming infected: for example, a cut has been contaminated with soil, faeces or a dirty blade, or fragments of material such as grit or glass which can be seen in the wound.

The wound has become infected: signs include swelling of the affected area, pus coming from the wound, redness spreading from the wound and increasing pain. The wound cannot be closed with a plaster, or it starts to open up when it moves.

The wound will create an unwelcome scar: for example, if it occurs on a prominent part of the casualty's face.

BRUISING

Bruises are bluish or purple-coloured patches that appear on the skin when tiny blood vessels (capillaries) break or burst underneath it.

The blood from the capillaries leak into the soft tissue under the skin causing the discolouration.

Over time this fades through shades of yellow or green.

Bruises often feel tender or swollen at first.

WHAT CAUSES BRUISING?

Bruising is caused by internal bleeding (under the skin) due to a person injuring themselves by, for example, falling over, walking into something or playing sports.

Some people are naturally more likely to bruise than others, for example, the elderly may bruise more easily because their skin is thinner and the tissue underneath is more fragile.

Treatment for bruises

Treat bruises, initially, by limiting the bleeding. You can do this by cooling the area with a cold compress (a flannel or cloth soaked in cold water) or an ice pack wrapped in a towel.

To make an ice pack, place ice cubes or a packet of frozen vegetables in a plastic bag and wrap them in a towel. Hold this over the affected area for at least 10 minutes.

Do not put the ice pack straight onto the skin as this will possibly cause further damage.

Most bruises will disappear after around two weeks.

If the bruise is still there after two weeks, you should recommend that your casualty see their GP.

INTERNAL BRUISING

Bruises don't just happen under the skin - they can also happen deeper in the body's tissues, organs and bones.

While the bleeding isn't visible, the bruises can cause swelling and pain.

You should recommend that your casualty seeks medical attention, or call for an ambulance if you feel the injury is of a serious nature, particularly if they have been involved in an accident.

NOSEBLEEDS

A common injury that is caused generally by a direct blow or sneezing. However, high blood pressure can also cause a sudden bleed with little warning.

If the blood is watery, then it could suggest a head injury, therefore making the incident far more serious i.e. possible skull fracture.

Treatment

- Sit the casualty down and lean them forward
- Ask them to pinch the soft part of the nose as they lean forward
- Apply this pressure for 10 minutes and then release slowly
  - Ask them to avoid rubbing or blowing their nose
  - If you are unable to stop the bleeding, ask them to repeat the pinching process for a further 10 minutes
    - If the bleeding continues then you will need to seek medical advice

If you suspect a head injury, then an ambulance must be summoned.

If the casualty is feeling faint or nausea you may consider sitting the casualty on the floor with their back supported. This could potentially prevent a fall.

SMALL SPLINTERS

A foreign body or object in first aid terms, relates to an object of any size that enters the body through many of its orifices, or penetrates the skin and is embedded.

You have to make a decision on whether you can remove it without having to seek medical help.

If a common embedded object such as a splinter is partly exposed, then it is acceptable to remove it with tweezers. First aid tweezers generally come in a sterile package. Washing grit away, under running water, can also be a useful treatment. If this won't remove the object, then the wound should be dressed with a sterile dressing, without putting direct pressure on the object, and then to seek medical attention.

However, for other objects such as glass or a fishing hook, they must be left in place and you should not attempt to remove it. Dress the wound appropriately and seek medical advice.

Animal and human bites are a relatively common type of injury. In most cases, the wound that results from an animal bite is minor and can be treated with simple first aid techniques.

DOG BITES

Dog bites typically cause a puncture wound (a narrow and deep hole) in the skin. They can also cause a laceration (a jagged wound or cut) and an abrasion (a scraped area of skin).

This is because dogs use their front teeth to "pin" their victim, and their other teeth to bite and pull at the surrounding skin.

CAT BITES

A cat bite is not as strong as a dog's, but their teeth are sharper and often cause very deep puncture wounds. A cat bite is capable of penetrating bones and joints. Lacerations and abrasions are less common, occurring in one-in-five cases.

HUMAN BITES

Most human bites are the result of a closed-fist injury, where one person punches another person in the teeth and cuts their hand. Typical symptoms include small cuts to the hand, and red, swollen and painful skin.

BITES AND STINGS continued

Toddlers often bite each other when playing together, but the resulting injuries are usually minor and do not usually pose a serious risk to their health.

General treatment

- **Make the area safe**
- **Reduce the risk of infection by wearing gloves**
- **Clean the wound immediately by running warm tap water over it for a couple of minutes**
- **Inspect the wound for embedded objects such as teeth and remove if you are able to**
- **Dry the wound and cover it with a sterile dressing**
- **Treat for shock**

When to seek medical advice:

You should seek immediate medical attention for all but minor dog or cat bites.

However, even some minor-looking cat bites can penetrate deeply and become infected.

Human bites have a much higher chance of causing infection, so always seek immediate medical attention before waiting for any symptoms of infection to appear.

Symptoms of infection

- **Redness and swelling around the wound. The wound becomes more painful**
- **Discharge from the wound**
- **Swollen lymph glands (nodes)**
- **A high temperature (fever) of 38°C (100.4°F) or above**
- **Shivers**

Always seek immediate medical attention if you or your child receives a bite to the following areas:

- **The hands**
- **The feet**
- **A joint, tendon or ligament**
- **The scalp or face**
- **The genitals**
- **The ears or nose**

Dial 999 immediately to request an ambulance if your child receives bite wounds to their head, neck or face. These types of wound can cause high amounts of blood loss, particularly in young children aged 10 or under and babies, and may therefore require emergency treatment.

If they have been bitten, the most important thing to do is to clean the wound immediately by running run warm tap water over the wound for 10 minutes.

In cases of serious bites, where a body part such as a finger or ear has been bitten off, you should wash the body part with tap water and place it in a plastic bag or a sealed container. Put the bag or container into a tub of iced water (but not frozen) to keep it cool, so that it can be transported to hospital. It may be possible to reattach the body part using reconstructive surgery.

Fortunately, in the seas around the UK, there are only a few types of marine creatures that sting.

These include weever fish, jellyfish, Portuguese man-of-war, sea urchins and stingrays. The symptoms and treatments for sea creature stings are all very similar. For the purposes of paediatric first aid, we will focus on weever fish and jellyfish.

WEEVER FISH

Weever fish have poisonous spines on their back and gills. Most people are stung on their feet by them after accidentally stepping on them.

Signs and symptoms

- Severe pain
- Itching
- Swelling (inflammation)
- Redness
- Numbness
- Tingling
- Nausea
- Vomiting
- Headache
- Joint ache
- Abdominal cramps
- Lightheadedness
- Temors (shaking)

If a person has a more serious reaction to a weever fish sting, they may experience:

- An abnormal heart rhythm (arrhythmia)
- Shortness of breath
- Weakness
- Paralysis
- Seizures (fits)
- A drop in blood pressure
- Episodes of unresponsiveness

Treatment

Seek medical assistance immediately.

To control the pain, the affected area should be immersed in hot water (as hot as can be tolerated) for between 30-90 minutes. This can be repeated if necessary. When the area has been numbed, be careful not to burn it with the hot water.

Thoroughly clean the wound using soap and water, before rinsing with fresh water. Do not cover the wound.

JELLYFISH

Jellyfish are mushroom-shaped creatures that have many long, thin tentacles on the underside of their bodies. The tentacles are covered with small poisonous sacs called nematocysts which, if touched, produce a nasty sting.

Jellyfish live in seas throughout the world and are found at a wide range of depths, although they often float near the surface. In recent years, during the warmer months, large swarms of jellyfish have become increasingly common in the seas around Europe, such as the Mediterranean.

Experts believe the increase in jellyfish numbers may be the result of increasingly warmer weather conditions combined with overfishing of their natural predators.

If you are stung by a jellyfish, you will experience some immediate symptoms such as:

- **Severe pain**
- **Itching**
- **A rash**
- **Raised welts (raised, circular areas on the skin)**

Other symptoms that you may have include:

- **Nausea**
- **Vomiting**
- **Diarrhoea**
- **Abdominal pain**
- **Muscle spasms**
- **Numbness**
- **Tingling**
- **Swollen lymph nodes**

(lymph nodes are small nodules that are found in several areas around the body, including in the groin and armpit)

In rare cases, a serious reaction to a jellyfish sting can result in breathing difficulties, coma or death.

When to seek medical advice

If someone has been stung by a jellyfish, seek immediate medical assistance by dialling 999 if they:

- **Are having problems breathing, or swallowing**
- **Have chest pain**
- **Have severe pain at the site of the sting**
- **Are very young or elderly**
- **Have been stung on a large area of the body or the face or the genitals**
- **There is severe pain, itchiness or inflammation (swelling) around the sting**

Treatment

Someone stung by a jellyfish should be treated out of the water. They should stay as still as possible while being treated because movement increases the risk of toxins being released into the body.

Any remaining tentacles should be removed using tweezers or the edge of a bank card (wear gloves if they're available). Soak the affected area in very warm water (as hot as can be tolerated) for at least 30 minutes – use hot flannels or towels if you can't soak it.

Vinegar is no longer recommended for treating jellyfish stings because it may make things worse by activating unfired stinging cells. The use of other substances, such as alcohol and baking soda, should also be avoided.

Ignore any advice you may have heard about urinating on the sting. It's unlikely to help and may make the situation worse.

Many insects sting as a defence mechanism by injecting venom into the skin.
In the UK, stinging insects include:

- **Bees** (honeybees and bumblebees)
- **Wasps**
- **Hornets**

Insect stings usually cause a swollen, red, raised mark to form on the skin. This is known as a weal.
The affected area will often be painful and itchy. This will usually last for a few days.

If you are stung by an insect, such as a wasp, the area around the sting will become inflamed
(swollen), go red and a raised mark (weal) will form. The affected area will often be quite painful
and itchy. This will usually last for a few days.

People who have an allergic reaction to an insect sting will experience more symptoms.
An allergic reaction occurs when the venom from the sting triggers the release of chemicals in the
body, such as histamine.

**Seek emergency medical treatment if, immediately after being stung, you experience any of the
following:**

- Swelling or itching anywhere else on your body
- A skin reaction anywhere else, particularly pale or flushed
  (red or blotchy) skin
- Wheezing, hoarseness or any difficulty breathing
- A headache
- Nausea, vomiting or diarrhoea
- A fast heart rate
- Dizziness or feeling faint
- Difficulty swallowing (dysphagia)
- A swollen face or mouth
- Confusion, anxiety or agitation

Treatment

Bee stings have a venomous sac attached. After you have been stung, the sting and the venomous sac will remain behind and the bee will die.

Wasps and hornets do not usually leave the sting behind and therefore could continue to sting you. If you have been stung and the wasp or hornet remains in the area, walk away calmly to avoid getting stung again.

Remove the sting immediately

As soon as you have been stung by an insect, you should remove the sting and the venomous sac. Do this by scraping it out with a hard edge, such as a bank card.

When removing the sting, be careful not to spread the venom further under your skin and that you do not puncture the venomous sac. Do not attempt to pinch the sting out with your fingers or a pair of tweezers, as you may spread the venom. If a child has been stung, an adult should remove the sting.

Basic treatment

To treat insect stings:

- **Wash the affected area with soap and water**
- **Put a cold flannel on the area**
- **Raise the part of the body that has been stung to prevent swelling**
- **Avoid scratching the area because it may become infected (see below)**
- **Keep children's fingernails short and clean**
- **Visit your GP if the redness and itching gets worse or does not clear up after a few days**

Snake bites

Snakes sometimes bite in self-defence if they are disturbed or provoked.

Adders, or vipers, are the only wild venomous snakes in the UK.

Adders sometimes bite without injecting any venom (toxins produced by the snake).

This is called a 'dry' bite and may cause:

Mild pain caused by the adder's teeth puncturing the skin, and anxiety.

If an adder injects venom when it bites it can cause more serious symptoms including:

- Swelling and redness in the area of the bite
- Nausea (feeling sick)
- Vomiting
- Faintness

Immediate action

If a snake bites you, or someone else, you should follow the advice listed below.

- Remain calm and do not panic. Snake bites, particularly those that occur in the UK, are rarely serious and very rarely fatal
- Try to remember the shape, size and colour of the snake
- Keep the part of your body that has been bitten as still as possible because this will prevent the venom spreading around your body. You may want to secure the bitten body part with a sling (a supportive bandage) or a splint (a rigid support that helps keep the body part stable). However, do not make the sling or splint so tight that it restricts your blood flow
- Remove any jewellery and watches from the bitten limb because they could cut into your skin if the limb swells. However, do not attempt to remove any clothing, such as trousers
- Seek immediate medical attention immediately

If you or someone else is bitten by a snake YOU SHOULD NEVER:

- Suck the venom out of the bite
- Cut the venom out of the bite wound with a knife or other instrument
- Rub anything into the wound
- Apply any tight bandage around the bitten limb to stop the spread of venom, such as a tourniquet or ligature